JA'NERA MITCHOM

The Ultimate Guide to Wavy, Curly & Coily Hair

Contents

1

Introduction

Embrace the natural texture of your hair. Your curls are unique and beautiful, just like you

Curly hair is one of the most complex hair types in the world today due to its unique texture, shape, and structure. You never know, on a daily basis, exactly what you are going to get. Caring for curly hair requires specialized knowledge and techniques to maintain its health, manageability, and natural beauty. This guide aims to provide you with a deeper understanding of your curly hair and equip you with the tools and strategies needed to care for it effectively at home. Whether you have wavy, curly, or coily hair, this comprehensive resource will empower you to embrace your curls with confidence and pride, ensuring they look and feel their best every day. From washing and conditioning to styling and maintenance, embark on a journey to discover the beauty of your natural curls and unlock their full potential with the insights and tips provided.

2

Understanding Curly Hair

Curly hair is like a fingerprint – uniquely yours and absolutely beautiful.

No two curls on one head of hair are the same, reflecting the beautiful diversity and individuality of curly hair. Each curl possesses its own unique characteristics, from its shape and size to its level of bounce and definition. But what determines the shape of a person's hair? According to a 2020 article, hair consists of two structures: the strand (or the hair shaft) itself, and the hair follicle. A 2017 study notes that the shape of the hair follicle determines the shape of a person's hair. Curly hair follicles are "S" shaped, indicating they possess two bends.[1] This distinctive "S" configuration is believed to be established during embryonic development and typically remains unchanged throughout life. However, hair follicles naturally undergo structural changes due to hormone changes,

---

[1] Rees, M. (2023, November 8). *What to know about different hair types and how to care for them.* https://www.medicalnewstoday.com/articles/hair-types

certain medications, and even age. Chemical treatments like hair relaxers or perms can also change the structure of hair follicles.

Understanding the science behind curly hair is also essential for effective hair care and styling. Along with hair structure, the porosity and elasticity of the hair can help determine what the hair needs and thus help determine product choice. These factors play a significant role in determining the most suitable hair care products and techniques for curly hair, ensuring optimal hydration, resilience, and manageability.

What is porosity?

Porosity refers to the hair's ability to absorb and retain moisture, influenced by factors such as the hair's cuticle condition and environmental exposure. Determining the porosity of hair is crucial for tailoring an effective hair care routine. One common method to assess porosity is the water test, where a strand of clean, dry hair is placed in a bowl of water. If the hair sinks quickly, it likely has high porosity, indicating that the cuticle is raised and absorbs moisture easily. If the hair floats in the middle of the water, it may have normal porosity, suggesting that the cuticle is intact and retains moisture adequately. If the hair remains on the surface of the water, it may have low porosity, meaning that the cuticle is tightly sealed and struggles to absorb moisture. Additionally, observing how quickly hair dries after washing or how well it absorbs hair care products can also provide insights into its porosity level.

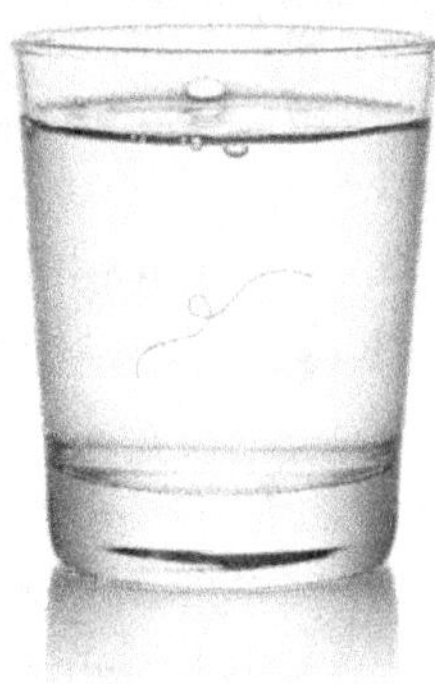

Hair Strand Porosity Test

What is elasticity?

Elasticity refers to the hair's ability to stretch and return to its original shape without breaking. Determining the elasticity of hair is essential for assessing its strength and resilience. One method to test hair elasticity is the stretch test, where a strand of clean, damp hair is gently stretched between the fingers.

Healthy hair should stretch and then return to its original length without breaking. If the hair stretches significantly and does not return to its original length, it may indicate low elasticity, suggesting that the hair is prone to breakage and damage. Conversely, if the hair breaks immediately without stretching, it may indicate high elasticity, indicating that the hair is overly stretched and weak. Observing how hair responds to manipulation, such as brushing or styling, can also provide insights into its elasticity.

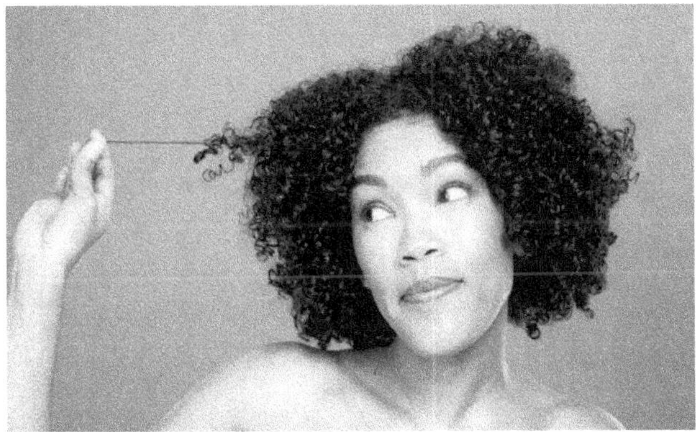

Understanding both the porosity and elasticity of the hair empowers individuals to choose suitable products, techniques, and hair care practices that cater to their curls' specific needs. By considering factors such as hydration, strength, flexibility, and overall health, individuals can tailor their hair care routines to achieve optimal results. Additionally, curl type is another crucial factor to consider when selecting products and techniques for hair care. In the next section, we will delve into the various curl types to provide a comprehensive understanding of how to best care for each type.

3

Types of Curly Hair

Your curls are your crown; wear them proudly

Although many people rely on the curly hair chart to determine their curl type, curly hair can essentially be categorized into just three types: wavy, curly, and coily. Wavy hair is characterized by loose waves that flow in an "S" pattern. Curly hair features tighter and more defined curls that form spirals or ringlets. Coily hair boasts the tightest and most compact curls, often forming intricate zigzag patterns and tight coils closer to the scalp. Each curl type requires specific care and styling techniques to enhance its natural beauty and maintain its health and vitality. Understanding the differences between wavy, curly, and coily hair types allows individuals to embrace their curls with confidence and tailor their hair care routine to meet their unique needs.

Hair Type Illustration

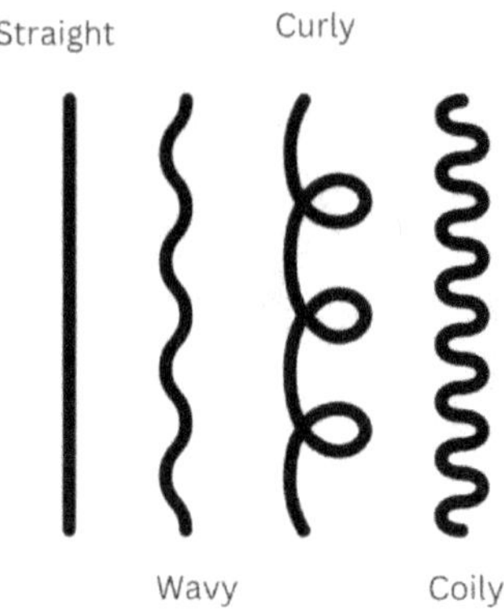

Wavy hair is known for its tendency to lose curl definition relatively quickly compared to tighter curl patterns, posing a challenge for those seeking to maintain defined curls for styling. Due to its looser wave pattern, wavy hair may struggle to hold onto curls or waves for extended periods, especially in humid or damp conditions. This can make it challenging to achieve and sustain the desired level of curl definition and volume when styling wavy hair. However, with the right products and styling techniques tailored to wavy hair's unique needs, individuals can enhance and prolong their waves, allowing for beautiful, effortless styling with minimal frizz and maximum hold.

Curly hair is more susceptible to frizz and dryness due to its unique structure, necessitating consistent hydration and the use of moisture-rich products to sustain its vibrancy and health. Common styling techniques like scrunching, diffusing, or plopping are frequently employed to accentuate curl definition and minimize frizz, ensuring that curls maintain buoyancy and manageability. While curly hair boasts more defined curls and bounce than wavy hair, it is typically considered less dense than its coily counterpart.

Coily hair, characterized by its dense and voluminous texture, is the most compact of the curly hair types. Individuals blessed with this curl pattern often find themselves dedicating entire days to the meticulous process of washing and styling their hair. The intricate coil structure of coily hair requires careful attention and patience to ensure thorough cleansing and effective styling. From detangling to defining each coil, the process demands time and effort to achieve desired results. Despite the labor-intensive nature of caring for coily hair, many embrace its abundant beauty and unique texture, finding joy and satisfaction in the journey of nurturing and styling their coils to perfection.

Understanding the unique characteristics of each curl type empowers individuals to customize their hair care routines and styling techniques accordingly, ensuring their curls' optimal health and beauty and celebrating their natural texture. In the upcoming section, we will delve into curated curly hair care routines tailored to address the distinct needs of each curl type, providing comprehensive guidance for nurturing and styling beautiful, healthy curls.

4

Curly Hair Care Routine

Curls are a journey, not a destination. Embrace every stage of your hair's evolution.

In the next sections, we will delve into comprehensive curly hair care routines designed to address the unique needs of each curl type. From wavy to coily hair, we'll provide tailored step-by-step guides for washing and styling, ensuring optimal results and curl definition. Additionally, we'll share valuable tips for refreshing curls between washes, helping you maintain their vibrancy, bounce, and definition throughout the week. Alongside practical advice for styling, we'll also tackle common concerns that often accompany curly hair, such as frizz, product buildup, dryness, shedding, and scalp issues. By addressing these concerns head-on and offering effective solutions, we aim to empower you to embrace and enhance your natural curls with confidence and ease. Get ready to embark on a journey to healthier, happier curls as we navigate the intricacies of curly hair care together.

Clarifying

For optimal curly hair care, we recommend clarifying your curls once a month to remove product buildup and other impurities effectively. This essential step helps to maintain a healthy scalp environment and ensures that your curls remain free from residue, allowing them to thrive and shine with vitality. By incorporating monthly clarifying treatments into your hair care routine, you can eliminate frizz, enhance curl definition, and promote overall hair health. This process of resetting your curls not only rejuvenates their natural bounce and texture but also prepares them for optimal styling, ensuring that your curls look and feel their best every day.

Deep Conditioning

Following a clarifying treatment, it's crucial to replenish moisture and nourishment to your curls by deep conditioning. Deep conditioning helps to restore hydration, softness, and elasticity to the hair strands, which may have been temporarily stripped during the clarifying process. This step is essential for maintaining the health and vitality of your curls, as well as preventing dryness, frizz, and breakage. Incorporating deep conditioning, after clarifying, into your hair care routine ensures that your curls remain strong, resilient, and beautifully moisturized, allowing them to thrive and maintain their natural vibrancy and bounce.

How often should you wash your curly hair?

To maintain the health and vitality of your curly hair, it's recommended to limit washing to no more than 1-2 times per week. Washing curly hair too frequently can strip away natural oils, leading to over-drying and potential damage to the hair strands. By reducing the frequency of washing, you allow your hair's natural oils to distribute evenly throughout the strands, helping to retain moisture and keeping your curls hydrated and resilient. Additionally, minimizing washing frequency can help preserve your curls' natural shape and definition, promoting overall hair health and minimizing the risk of frizz and breakage. Embracing a gentle washing routine tailored to your curls' needs ensures they remain vibrant, bouncy, and full of life.

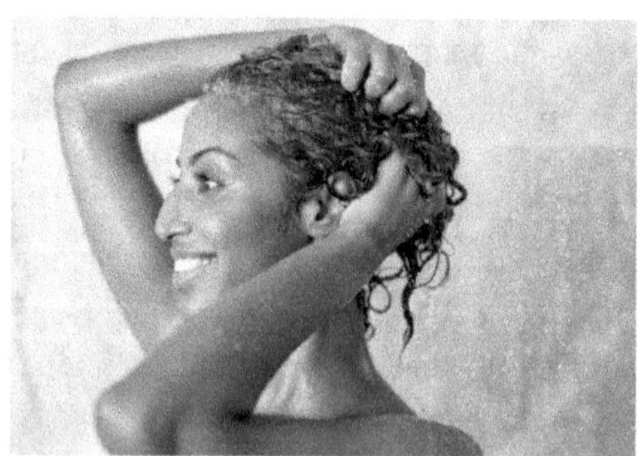

Step-by-Step Guide for Washing & Styling

Wavy Hair

Here's a step-by-step guide for washing, conditioning, and styling wavy hair:

1. **Wash**: Wet your hair thoroughly and wash it twice using a lightweight moisture shampoo. Focus on the scalp, massaging gently to remove dirt and buildup.
2. **Condition**: Apply a lightweight moisture conditioner from mid-lengths to ends, ensuring thorough coverage. Leave the conditioner on for a few minutes to allow it to penetrate the hair shaft.
3. **Detangle**: While the conditioner is still in your hair, use a detangling brush to gently detangle your hair, starting from the ends and working your way up to the roots.
4. **Rinse**: Rinse the conditioner completely with lukewarm water, being careful not to wring out the water.
5. **Product Application**: While your hair is still soaking wet, apply the first styling product evenly throughout. Then, divide your hair into sections and apply the second product in each section, adding more of the first product or water as needed. Scrunch each section as you go to encourage curl formation.
6. **Remove Excess Water**: Use a microfiber towel, cotton cloth, or T-shirt to gently scrunch out excess water from your hair, being careful not to disrupt the curl pattern.
7. **Drying**: Allow your hair to air dry for a natural look, or

use a diffuser on low heat to speed up the drying process and add volume to your waves. Avoid touching your curls while they dry to minimize frizz.

Following these steps will help you maintain healthy, hydrated, wavy hair and enhance the beauty and definition of your natural waves.

Curly Hair

Here's a step-by-step guide for washing and conditioning curly hair:

1. **Wash**: Wet your hair thoroughly and wash it twice using a moisture shampoo. Focus on the scalp, massaging gently to remove dirt and buildup while not stripping the hair of its natural oils
2. **Condition**: Apply a moisture conditioner generously from mid-lengths to ends, ensuring thorough coverage. Leave the conditioner on for a few minutes to allow it to penetrate the hair shaft and provide hydration.
3. **Detangle**: While the conditioner is still in your hair, use a detangling brush to gently detangle your curls, starting from the ends and working your way up to the roots. This helps to minimize breakage and tangles.
4. **Rinse**: Rinse the conditioner completely with lukewarm water, being careful not to wring out the water, as hair must be soaking wet for product application.
5. **Product Application**: While your hair is still soaking wet, apply the first styling product evenly throughout. Then, divide your hair into sections and apply the second

product in each section, adding more of the first product or water as needed. For elongated curls, brush products through to elongate curls and smooth cuticles. For volume, scrunch each section as you go to encourage curl formation.

6. **Remove Excess Water**: Use a microfiber towel, cotton cloth, or T-shirt to gently squeeze out excess water from your hair. Scrunch the hair upwards to enhance volume. For an elongated finish, wrap the towel around your curls and gently squeeze to elongate them.

7. **Drying:** Allow your hair to air dry for a natural look, or use a diffuser on low heat to speed up the drying process while enhancing volume. Avoid touching your curls while they dry to minimize frizz.

Following these steps will help you maintain hydrated, defined curls while preventing frizz and maximizing volume.

Techniques to Refresh Wavy/Curly Hair

To refresh curls in between washes for wavy or curly hair, begin by lightly dampening the hair with water, ensuring not to soak it entirely. Then, apply a small amount of foam or mousse to the damp hair, scrunching it in to encourage curl formation and revive bounce. Alternatively, opt for a pea-sized amount of conditioner or leave-in conditioner, applying it to the hair in sections using the praying hands method to ensure even distribution. After applying the product, gently scrunch the hair to reactivate the curls. Finally, choose to either diffuse the hair on low heat or allow it to air dry naturally. These techniques help to revive and redefine curls, extending the time between washes while maintaining the hair's moisture and texture.

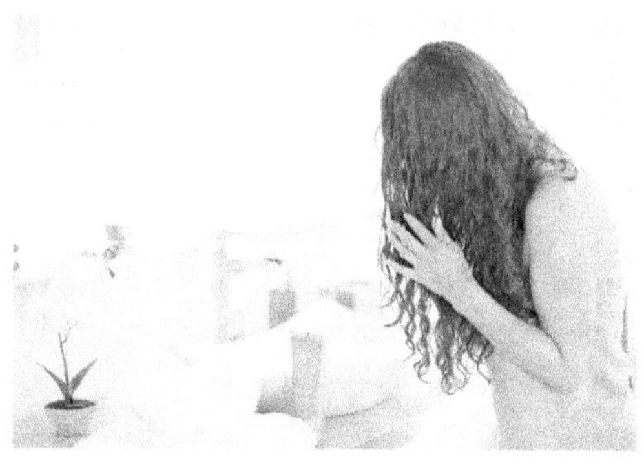

Coily Hair

Here's a step-by-step guide for washing and conditioning coily hair:

1. **Wash**: Wet your hair thoroughly and wash it twice using a moisture shampoo. Focus on the scalp, massaging gently to remove dirt and buildup while maintaining the hair's natural oils.
2. **Condition**: Apply a moisture conditioner generously

from roots to ends, ensuring thorough coverage. Leave the conditioner on for several minutes to allow it to penetrate the hair shaft deeply and provide maximum hydration.

3. **Detangle**: While the conditioner is still in your hair, use a detangling brush to gently detangle your coils, starting from the ends and working your way up to the roots. This helps minimize breakage and tangles.

4. **Rinse**: Rinse the conditioner completely with lukewarm water, being careful not to wring out the water, as hair must be soaking wet for product application.

5. **Product Application**: While your hair is still soaking wet, apply the first styling product thoroughly throughout your hair in sections, ensuring that each strand is covered from root to end.

6. **Add More Water**: If needed, add more water to your hair without soaking it completely. This helps to activate the styling products and encourages curl definition.

7. **Second Product Application:** Divide your hair into sections and apply the second product in each section, adding more of the first product or water as needed. Brush the products through to elongate curls and smooth cuticles for a defined look.

8. **Drying**: Allow your hair to air dry, or use a diffuser on low heat to set the curls. To prevent frizz, avoid touching your hair until it is completely dry to prevent frizz. Once dry, you can fluff or style your coils as desired.

Following these steps will help you maintain hydrated, defined coils while preventing frizz and maximizing curl definition and your style should last for at least 7 days or until your next wash day.

Techniques to Avoid for Coily Hair

Avoiding the **LOC** (Liquid, Oil, Cream) method and **co-washing** can be beneficial for individuals with coily hair, as these techniques may not provide adequate moisture and cleansing for this hair type. While the LOC method is popular for sealing in moisture, the heavy use of oils and creams can lead to product buildup, weighing down coily hair and hindering curl definition. Instead, opt for lightweight, water-based gels that provide hydration without leaving a greasy residue. Additionally, co-washing, or using conditioner alone to cleanse the hair, may not effectively remove dirt, sweat, and product buildup from coily hair, which is prone to trapping impurities due to its dense texture. Instead, incorporate a gentle, sulfate-free shampoo into your hair care routine to ensure thorough cleansing while maintaining moisture balance. By avoiding the LOC method and co-washing, individuals with coily hair can maintain clean, hydrated strands and optimize their curl definition and overall hair health.

Techniques to Refresh Coily Hair

While we don't recommend co-washing as a replacement for weekly shampoos, it can be an effective technique to refresh coily hair in between washes, provided it's followed up with a thorough shampoo on the next wash day. Co-washing helps to maintain moisture and set a good foundation for styling by gently cleansing the hair without stripping away natural oils. After co-washing, consider adding a lightweight gel to enhance curl definition and longevity. This combination of co-washing and lightweight styling products can extend the life of your wash-and-go, keeping your coily hair hydrated and looking its best for an additional 3-4 days.

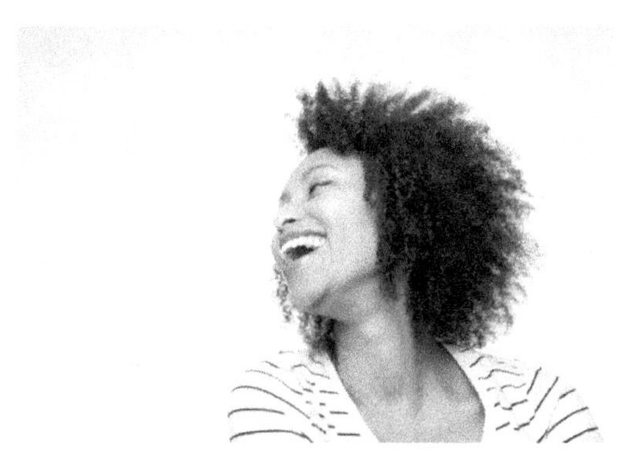

With the comprehensive washing, styling, and refreshing guide provided above, you're well-equipped to embark on a journey toward achieving healthy, beautiful curls that exude confidence and radiance. By incorporating the recommended techniques into your hair care routine, from selecting the right products to mastering effective styling and refreshing methods, you're nurturing your curls to their fullest potential. In the upcoming section, we'll delve deeper into advanced styling techniques, including expert insights on product application, diffusing, and plopping. These techniques will serve as invaluable tools to elevate your curls to the next level, enabling you to unlock their true beauty and embrace a newfound sense of curl empower-ment. Get ready to witness your curls flourishing like never before as we explore the secrets to achieving stunning, head-turning curls that reflect your unique style and personality.

5

Styling Tips & Techniques

Embrace the chaos of curls. There's beauty in every twist and turn

Next up, we will delve into a range of styling techniques tailored specifically for wavy, curly, and coily hair types. From enhancing natural waves to defining curls and coils, we'll explore a variety of methods and tips to help you achieve your desired look. Whether you're aiming for loose beachy waves, defined coils, or voluminous curls, we've got you covered. Get ready to unlock the secrets to styling your unique hair texture with confidence and flair. Let's dive in and discover the endless possibilities for embracing and enhancing your waves, curls, and coils.

Product Application

Product application plays a crucial role in achieving optimal styling results and enhancing curl definition. The way you apply products to your hair can greatly impact how well your curls hold their shape, maintain moisture, and resist frizz throughout the day. Whether you're using styling gel or mousse, it's essential to distribute the product evenly from root to tip, ensuring that each strand is coated thoroughly. Additionally, applying products in sections and using techniques like scrunching or raking can help encourage curl formation and maximize product absorption. By mastering the art of product application, you can unleash the full potential of your curls and achieve the stunning, long-lasting results you desire.

The cornerstone of effective product application lies in hydration, often in the form of water. Ensuring maximum hydration is crucial when applying styling products, as it facilitates even distribution and helps prevent frizz. Before applying any products, it's essential to start with thoroughly wet hair, as this primes the hair for optimal product absorption. Spritzing water can help replenish moisture and prepare the hair for styling. By prioritizing hydration during product application, you set the stage for well-defined, frizz-free curls that retain their shape and vitality throughout the day.

Working in sections is also a key technique for achieving even distribution of product throughout your hair. By dividing your hair into manageable sections, you can focus on applying the product thoroughly and evenly, ensuring that each strand receives the hydration and styling benefits it needs. This method allows you to take your time and pay attention to each section, reducing the risk of missing spots or applying too much product in one area. Regardless of the product you are using, working in sections helps maximize product absorption and ensures that your curls are consistently well-defined and moisturized from root to tip. Incorporating this technique into your styling routine can elevate your results and leave you with beautifully styled, frizz-free curls that last.

Product Selection

Selecting the appropriate products for your curls is paramount to achieving the desired appearance and health of your locks, whether you're aiming for enhanced curl definition or added volume. Various factors such as porosity, elasticity, environmental conditions, hormonal changes, age, and the current condition of your hair and scalp also play significant roles in selecting the most suitable product. Regardless of your curl type, opt for products that are free of sulfates, silicones, and parabens. These ingredients can strip the hair of its natural oils and lead to dryness and damage over time. Additionally, it's advisable to steer clear of leave-ins, oils, and heavy creams as primary styling products, as they tend to weigh down the curls and create a barrier that blocks moisture absorption, ultimately exacerbating frizz. Instead, opt for lightweight, water-based styling products that provide hydration and hold without compromising the natural bounce and movement of your curls. By making informed choices about your hair care products, you can maintain the vibrancy and vitality of your curls while achieving your desired hairstyle with ease.

Product Combinations

Styling your curls with a strategic combination of products can make a significant difference in achieving your desired look. For those seeking enhanced definition and long-lasting results, layering a lightweight gel underneath a heavier gel can be highly effective. The lightweight gel provides initial hold and moisture, while the heavier gel seals in the shape and creates a cast that helps your curls maintain their form throughout the day. This combination ensures that your curls remain defined and frizz-free for an extended period.

Alternatively, if you're aiming to add volume to your curls while maintaining definition, pairing a lightweight gel with a foam or mousse can yield impressive results. The lightweight gel provides initial hold and moisture, while the foam or mousse adds volume and texture, resulting in fuller-looking curls with enhanced definition. This combination strikes the perfect balance between volume and definition, giving your curls a voluminous yet well-defined appearance.

For those who prefer maximum volume without sacrificing definition, opting for a single product, such as a foam, mousse, or lightweight gel, can provide the desired results. While this approach may offer immediate volume, it's important to note that the results may not last as long compared to layering products. Nonetheless, using a single product can still yield impressive volume and bounce, perfect for those looking to make a statement with their curls. By experimenting with different product combinations and techniques, you can discover the perfect styling routine that meets your unique curl needs and preferences.

Let's address the common concern of the dreaded cast. Contrary to popular belief, setting your curls with products that will create a cast is actually beneficial. This cast, formed by certain styling products as they dry, is instrumental in ensuring the success and longevity of your curls. It provides structure and definition, helping your curls maintain their shape throughout the day. Once your hair is fully dry, breaking the cast is simple – just use your favorite oil to gently scrunch or fluff your curls. This process reveals soft, fluffy curls that are primed and ready to be showcased to the world, boasting enhanced definition and volume. Embracing the cast is a straightforward yet effective technique for achieving stunning, long-lasting curls that make a statement wherever you go.

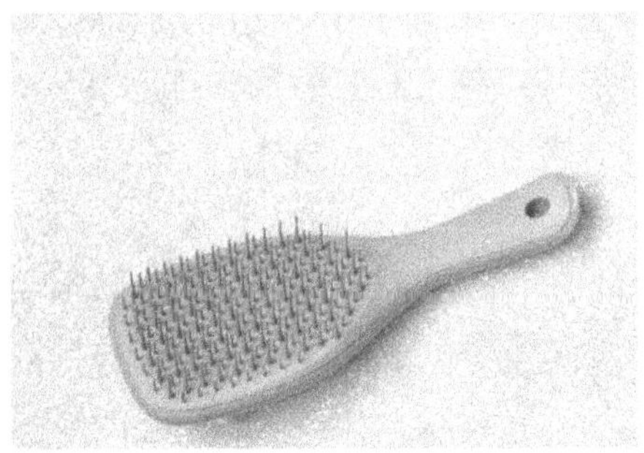

Detangling

Detangling curly hair can be a daunting task, especially considering the varying densities of curls. To tackle this challenge effectively, it's beneficial to divide your hair into manageable sections, typically four for most curly hair types and five for coily hair. This segmentation allows you to focus on one area at a time, making the detangling process more manageable. As you work through each section, clip away the already detangled hair to prevent re-tangling. Begin detangling from the ends of your hair, gently working your way up to the scalp. This approach helps to minimize damage and breakage while ensuring that all tangles are effectively eliminated. By following these tips and techniques, detangling curly hair becomes a smoother and less overwhelming experience, resulting in healthier, more manageable curls.

Diffusing

Diffusing your curls is not only a fantastic method for adding volume, but it can also be incredibly beneficial in setting your hair to air dry and assisting in breaking the cast once dry. By using a diffuser attachment on your hair dryer, you can gently dry your curls while simultaneously enhancing their natural volume and texture. This process helps to distribute airflow evenly, minimizing frizz and maintaining the integrity of your curls. Additionally, diffusing can aid in setting your hair to air dry by accelerating the drying process without sacrificing curl definition. Incorporating diffusing into your styling routine is a versatile and effective way to achieve beautiful, long-lasting curls with added volume and definition.

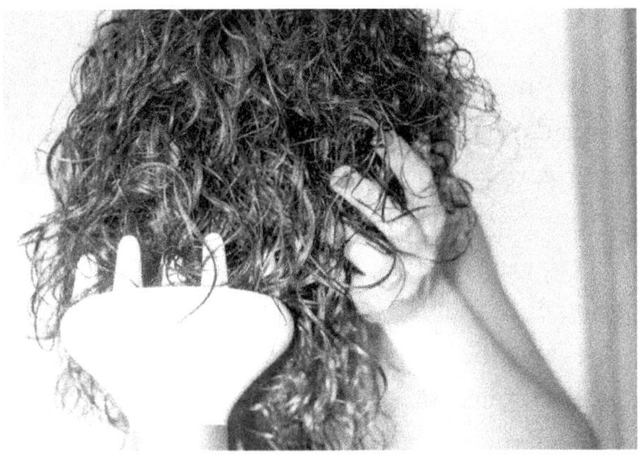

Techniques

For less volume and more definition - all curl types

When it comes to diffusing techniques suitable for all hair types, aiming for less volume and more definition is achievable with a strategic approach. Begin by setting your hair dryer on low to medium heat and a low airflow setting. With the diffuser attachment, gently hover over your curls to evenly distribute heat and product, effectively setting a cast that enhances curl definition. Once the cast is established, you have the option to either air dry or utilize a hooded dryer to complete the drying process. Once your hair is fully dry, simply scrunch or fluff your curls to remove the cast, revealing beautifully defined curls with minimal volume.

For those with coily hair, we recommend incorporating the praying hands method to break the cast and maintain curl definition. After diffusing to set the cast, once your hair is completely dry, gently run your hands down the length of your curls in a praying motion to loosen the cast and encourage softness and movement. This technique helps to minimize frizz while preserving the integrity of your coils. By integrating these diffusing techniques into your styling routine, you can achieve the perfect balance of volume and definition for your unique hair texture, whether you prefer a natural look or enhanced curl definition.

For volume - wavy/curly hair

When aiming to enhance volume for wavy or curly hair, utilizing a strategic diffusing technique can make all the difference. Begin by hovering the diffuser over your hair to set a cast, ensuring even distribution of product and heat. Once the cast is established, divide your hair into sections and gently scrunch the curls upward into the diffuser. This technique helps to amplify volume while maintaining curl definition. For an extra boost of volume, flip your hair upside down and diffuse from underneath. This method encourages lift at the roots and adds overall fullness to your hair. By incorporating these diffusing techniques into your styling routine, you can achieve voluminous, bouncy curls that command attention and leave you feeling confident all day long.

Diffusing for volume for coily hair

For coily hair seeking a more voluminous appearance, we recommend a strategic product combination to achieve the desired effect. Rather than using scrunching and diffusing techniques, opting for a layered approach with specific products can elevate volume while maintaining curl definition. We suggest using a combination of gel layered with a foam or mousse. The gel provides the necessary hold and moisture to shape and define the coils, while the foam adds volume and texture, resulting in fuller-looking coils with enhanced bounce and vitality. This product pairing offers a balanced and effective method for achieving maximum volume without sacrificing curl definition. By incorporating this product choice combination into your styling routine, you can enjoy voluminous and well-defined coily hair that commands attention with its natural beauty and texture.

Plopping

Plopping, when executed correctly, can be a fantastic technique for enhancing volume and defining curls, especially for those with wavy or curly hair. This method involves wrapping damp hair in a T-shirt or microfiber towel to encourage natural curl formation and reduce frizz while allowing the hair to dry. We recommend plopping after applying styling products to maximize hydration and ensure even product distribution throughout the hair. By plopping with styling products already in place, you can capitalize on the moisture-retaining properties of the fabric, allowing your curls to absorb the product more effectively and maintain their shape as they dry. Incorporating plopping into your styling routine can result in beautifully voluminous and defined curls that last throughout the day.

To plop your hair effectively, start with freshly washed and conditioned hair. After applying your styling products, lay a T-shirt or microfiber towel flat on a surface, with the sleeves closest to you. Lower your head forward and carefully lower your hair onto the center of the fabric, allowing your curls to gather towards the crown of your head naturally. Next, fold the bottom of the towel or T-shirt over the back of your head, covering your hair completely. Secure the fabric by tying or twisting the sleeves around the front of your head, creating a turban-like shape. Leave your hair plopped for about 10-30 minutes, depending on your hair thickness and desired level of moisture retention. Once time is up, gently unwrap the fabric and allow your hair to air dry, or use a diffuser on low heat to finish drying. Plopping helps enhance curl definition and reduce frizz, leaving you with beautifully styled curls ready to take on the day.

With the right combination of styling products, product application techniques, and styling methods, such as diffusing or plopping, you have all the tools needed to achieve the perfect look for your curls, no matter the occasion. By selecting the appropriate products tailored to your hair type and desired outcome and applying them with precision to ensure even distribution, you can lay the foundation for stunning, well-defined curls. Whether you choose to enhance volume and definition with diffusing, or encourage natural curl formation with plopping, or opt for a more defined look, these styling techniques can elevate your curls to new heights. With a bit of experimentation and practice, you'll discover the ideal routine that leaves your curls looking and feeling their best, ready to shine at any event or occasion.

Techniques to Approach with Caution for Coily Hair

Blow Dryer Stretching for Coily Hair

Using a blow dryer to stretch coily hair is generally discouraged due to the potential risk of losing the natural curl pattern. The heat from the blow dryer can cause the hair to become overly stretched, leading to a looser curl or straightening effect over time. Additionally, regularly slicking back the hair using gel can also contribute to curl loss, particularly in the area where the gel is applied. This is a common issue among individuals with natural hair who may not use heat styling tools but still experience curl loss, especially in the front sections of their hair, where manipulation and styling are most frequent. Opting for gentler styling methods and products specifically designed for coily hair can help preserve the natural curl pattern and maintain healthy, vibrant curls without risking damage or loss.

Protective Styling for Coily Hair

Protective styles have become a staple in the curly hair community, potentially offering a way to promote hair growth and create the illusion of length. While these styles are beneficial, it's crucial to remember that they should not replace regular trims, as trimming is the only way to eliminate split ends and encourage healthy hair growth. Additionally, it's wise to steer clear of braids as a protective style, as the tension from braiding can lead to hair loss and breakage over time. Furthermore, when opting for protective styles, it's best to avoid putting them on hair that has been stretched from blow drying, as this can result in potential curl loss over time. By utilizing protective styles safely and incorporating regular trims, individuals can maintain healthy curls and support overall hair health.

6

Curly Hair Cuts

Life is too short to have boring hair. Embrace your curls and let them shine!

Maintaining healthy curly hair requires regular maintenance, including getting regular haircuts or trims every 3-4 months, regardless of the curl type. These trims are essential for eliminating dead ends and preventing split ends from traveling up the hair shaft, which can lead to further damage and breakage. By scheduling regular trims, you're not only preserving the overall health of your curls but also promoting optimal growth and length retention. Additionally, trims allow for the removal of any damaged or weakened areas, ensuring that your curls remain vibrant, bouncy, and full of life.

Hair cutting for curly hair requires a specialized approach that considers the unique characteristics and behaviors of curls. Unlike straight hair, curls have varying levels of elasticity, density, and curl pattern, which must be considered when determining the most suitable haircut. Curly hair tends to shrink when dry, so it's essential to cut the hair in its dry and natural state to ensure accuracy and precision. Additionally, cutting curly hair in its natural state allows the stylist to see how the curls will fall and react, resulting in a more tailored and flattering haircut. Layering techniques are often used to add dimension and shape to curly hair, while avoiding excessive bulk and maintaining curl definition. A skilled stylist will understand the importance of customizing the haircut to complement the client's curl pattern, face shape, and personal style, ultimately creating a haircut that enhances the natural beauty of the curls and celebrates their unique texture.

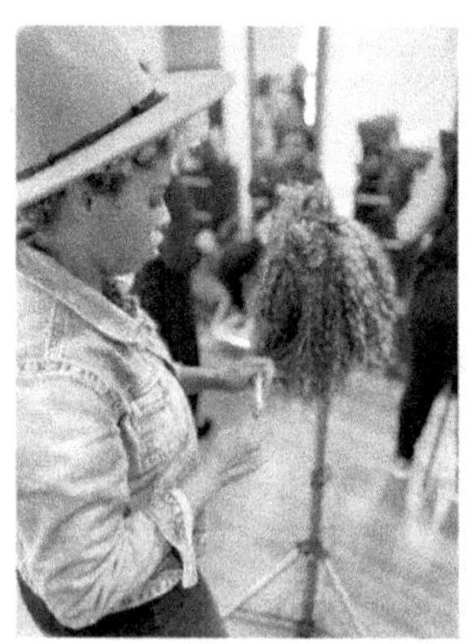

Locating a Curly Hair Specialist

When choosing a curly hair stylist, it's crucial to consider a few key factors to ensure you find the right match for your unique curls. One important aspect is to examine their social media platforms, particularly Instagram, for photos of clients with similar hair types to yours. This allows you to gauge the stylist's experience and skill level in working with curly hair and see if their previous clients' results align with your desired outcome. Additionally, look for evidence of ongoing education or certifications in curly hair-cutting techniques. This demonstrates a commitment to staying updated on the latest trends and methods for caring for and styling curly hair. By carefully assessing these factors, you can select a curly hair stylist who understands your specific needs and can provide personalized, high-quality service to help you achieve the curls of your dreams.

Communicating With Your Hair Stylist

When attending a haircut appointment for your curly hair, effective communication with your stylist is key to achieving the best results. Start by being clear and specific about your curl type, texture, and any particular concerns or goals you have for your hair. Providing visual references, such as pictures or examples of hairstyles you admire, can also help ensure you and your stylist are on the same page. During the appointment, don't hesitate to ask questions or voice any concerns you may have about the haircut process or the recommended styling techniques. Remember that your stylist is there to help you achieve your desired look, so open and honest communication is essential. Additionally, trust your instincts and speak up if you feel uncomfortable or unsure about any aspect of the haircut. By effectively communicating your needs and preferences, you can work collaboratively with your stylist to create a hairstyle that complements your curls and enhances their natural beauty.

When you have curly hair, it's essential to advocate for yourself when it comes to your hair. Embracing your natural curls means understanding their unique needs and communicating them effectively to hairstylists and other professionals. Whether requesting specific products or techniques that work best for your curl type, expressing concerns about potential damage or frizz, or simply asserting your preferences and boundaries, speaking up is key to ensuring that your curls are treated with the care and respect they deserve. By advocating for yourself and your curls, you empower yourself to make informed decisions and cultivate a positive relationship with your hairstylist. Remember, your curls are a beautiful expression of your identity, and advocating for them is a powerful act of self-love and self-expression.

By prioritizing regular haircuts and seeking a knowledgeable stylist who is well-versed in the unique needs and challenges of curly hair, we establish a strong foundation for success in our curly hair care journey. Additionally, advocating for ourselves and communicating our specific hair concerns and preferences to our stylist empowers us to receive personalized care and guidance tailored to our individual needs. Through this proactive approach, we not only ensure the health and vitality of our curls but also foster a sense of confidence and empowerment in embracing our natural texture. By taking ownership of our curly hair care routine and advocating for the expertise and support we deserve, we set ourselves up for long-term success and satisfaction with our curls.

7

Common Curly Hair Concerns

Curls are a gift; embrace them with gratitude.

In this section, we'll outline the common issues that individuals with curly hair frequently encounter, spanning a range of concerns from frizz and dehydration to shedding, hormonal changes, and scalp issues. By acknowledging and addressing these common challenges, individuals with curly hair can better navigate their hair care journey and achieve healthier, more resilient curls.

Frizz

Frizz is undeniably one of the most prevalent concerns for individuals with curly hair. Various factors, including weather conditions, product selection, and product buildup, contribute significantly to the ongoing battle against frizz. Humidity, in particular, tends to lead to frizz by causing the hair strands to swell and lose moisture, resulting in a frizzy appearance. Moreover, using the wrong products or failing to cleanse the hair adequately can lead to product buildup, which further exacerbates frizz. To combat frizz, curly-haired individuals must adopt a hair care routine tailored to their specific needs, incorporating moisture-rich shampoos and conditioners, regular cleansing, and proper styling product choices. By addressing these factors, individuals can effectively manage frizz and maintain beautifully defined curls.

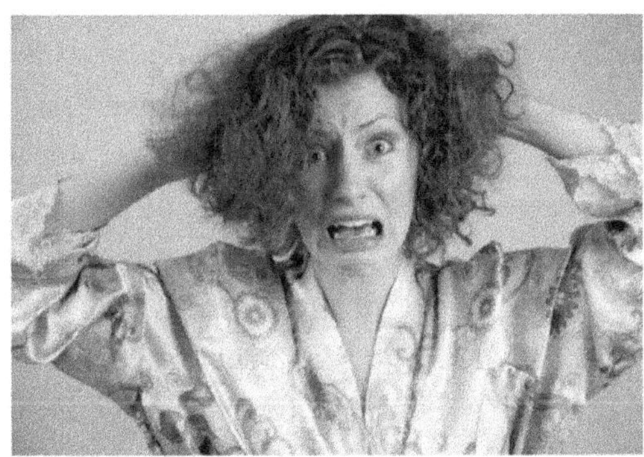

Dehydrated Hair

Dehydration is a prevalent concern for individuals with curly hair, as the natural oils produced by the scalp have difficulty reaching the lengths of the hair strands due to their unique structure. To address this issue, it's crucial to incorporate hydrating shampoos and conditioners specifically formulated for curly hair into your hair care routine. These products work to infuse moisture into the hair strands, leaving them feeling soft, supple, and hydrated. Additionally, regular monthly deep conditioning treatments can provide an extra boost of hydration and nourishment, helping to combat dehydration and keep curls looking healthy and vibrant.

On the flip side, it's important to be mindful of the potential for protein overload, which can also contribute to dehydration in curly hair. While protein is essential for maintaining the strength and structure of the hair, excessive use of protein-based products or treatments can lead to dryness and brittleness. To prevent protein overload and dehydration, it's essential to strike a balance between protein and moisture in your hair care regimen. Incorporating protein treatments in moderation and ensuring adequate hydration through deep conditioning can help maintain your curls' optimal health and hydration, keeping them looking their best.

Scalp Issues

While any scalp issues should be addressed by a dermatologist for proper diagnosis and treatment, it's important to note that proper drying techniques are also essential for maintaining scalp and hair health, especially when air drying curly hair. Before going to bed or putting your curls up in a pineapple or ponytail, ensure that both your hair and scalp are completely dry. This precaution helps to prevent the risk of mold and mildew formation on the scalp and hair, which can occur when moisture is trapped against the scalp for an extended period. While it may seem unlikely, this phenomenon can indeed happen, leading to unpleasant scalp conditions and potential hair damage. By prioritizing thorough drying before styling or resting, you can help safeguard the health and integrity of your scalp and curls.

Shedding

Hair shedding is a natural phenomenon. On average, it's normal to shed about 50 to 100 hairs per day. This shedding is part of the hair growth cycle, where old hairs are shed to make way for new ones. However, for those with curly hair, shed hair tends to become trapped within the curls, making it more noticeable. If you notice that your curls are shedding more than usual, it's important to address this with a trichologist or dermatologist. Excessive shedding can be a sign of various factors, including stress, hormonal changes, or underlying health conditions. Seeking professional advice will help determine the cause of increased shedding and allow for appropriate guidance and treatment to maintain the health and vitality of your curls.

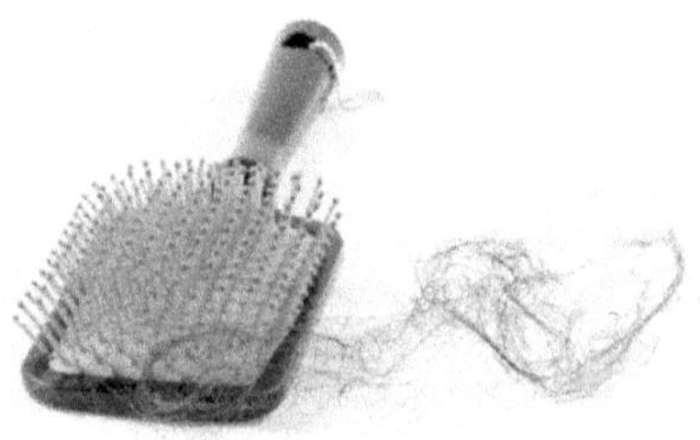

Hormonal Changes

Hormonal changes, such as those experienced during puberty, aging, and pregnancy, can have a significant impact on the texture and density of curls over time. During puberty, fluctuations in hormone levels can lead to alterations in hair texture, potentially causing curls to become more pronounced or undergo changes in density. Similarly, as individuals age, hormonal shifts can result in shifts in curl pattern and overall hair thickness. Pregnancy is another factor that can influence hair texture, with many women experiencing changes in curl pattern and density due to hormonal fluctuations during and after childbirth. These hormonal changes underscore the importance of adapting hair care routines to meet the evolving needs of one's curls throughout different stages of life.

Heat Styling

Embracing the versatility of our curly hair is undoubtedly one of its most cherished aspects. However, it's crucial to acknowledge the potential impact of heat styling, such as blowouts and flat ironing, on our natural curls. Regular exposure to high temperatures can gradually loosen the curl pattern, resulting in less defined curls or even straightened strands over time. To minimize these effects, it's essential to take proactive measures to protect our curls. One effective strategy is to incorporate products with heat protection properties into our styling routine, creating a protective barrier that shields the hair from heat damage. Additionally, opting for lower temperatures on our straighteners or curling irons can help mitigate the stress on our curls while still achieving desired styles. Furthermore, considering the frequency of heat styling and reducing its occurrence can also help preserve the integrity of our natural curl pattern. By implementing these precautionary steps and being mindful of our heat styling habits, we can maintain the versatility of our curly hair while safeguarding its health and vitality for the long term.

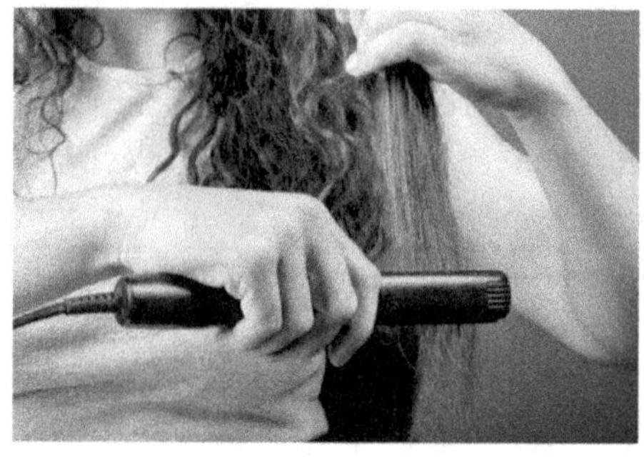

By confronting these common issues head-on, we empower ourselves to tailor our hair care routines to effectively address them, ultimately leading to healthier, more resilient curly hair. Whether it's implementing strategies to combat frizz, ensuring adequate hydration to prevent dryness, or adapting our routines to accommodate hormonal changes and scalp issues, proactive measures can make a significant difference in the overall health and appearance of our curls. By understanding the unique needs of curly hair and incorporating targeted solutions into our daily regimen, we can achieve the vibrant, well-nourished curls we desire. Embracing these challenges as opportunities for growth and learning allows us to cultivate a hair care routine that not only addresses current concerns but also sets the foundation for long-term hair health and confidence.

8

Lifestyle Tips

Curly hair is not a trend; it's a lifestyle

For many individuals with curly hair, lifestyle factors like nighttime care and exercise play significant roles in their daily routines. Finding effective ways to manage these influences becomes essential for maintaining healthy and vibrant curls throughout the day. By incorporating strategies to address these lifestyle factors, curly-haired individuals can better preserve their natural texture and ensure their hair looks its best despite the challenges of daily life.

Nighttime Care

Establishing a nighttime care routine is essential for maintaining the health and appearance of curly hair while ensuring minimal frizz and disruption to the natural curl pattern. One effective practice is sleeping with a satin bonnet or using a satin pillowcase. Satin's smooth texture helps reduce friction between the hair and the surface, preventing frizz and break-

45

age caused by rubbing against cotton or other rough fabrics. Additionally, satin helps retain moisture in the hair, preserving hydration and minimizing dryness overnight.

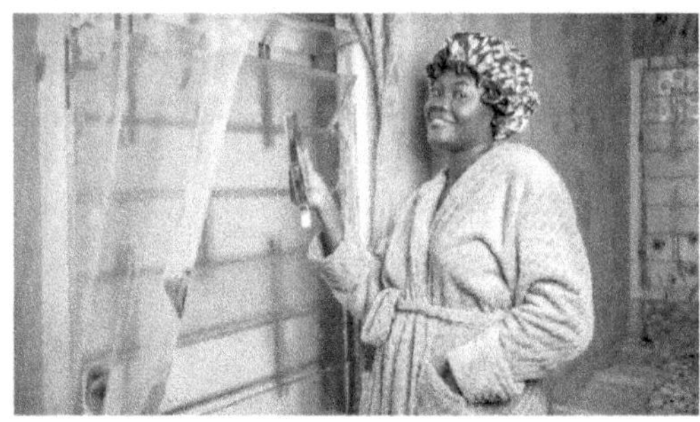

For those with curly hair, the pineapple method is a popular technique for preserving curls while sleeping. To pineapple, gather the hair loosely at the crown of the head and secure it with a scrunchie or satin hair tie. This technique helps prevent flattening of the curls and minimizes tangling, allowing you to wake up with refreshed, bouncy curls in the morning. However, it's essential to note that pineapple may not be suitable for all curl types. While it works well for curly hair, it may not be ideal for wavy or coily hair types, as it could potentially cause the curls to stretch or become misshapen.

Exercise

Caring for curly hair, especially for individuals who lead an active lifestyle and regularly engage in exercise, requires specific strategies to maintain the health and appearance of the curls. One effective method for preserving curls during workouts is pineappling. This technique involves loosely gathering the hair at the top of the head and securing it with a scrunchie or satin hair tie. Pineappling helps prevent friction and tangling, minimizing the risk of frizz and preserving the integrity of the curls while exercising.

For individuals with wavy or coily hair, braiding can be a beneficial alternative to pineappling. Braiding the hair before exercising helps prevent excessive movement and tangling, keeping the curls contained and protected during physical activity. Additionally, once unraveled, braids can create beautiful waves or coils, providing a stylish and effortless post-workout hairstyle.

After exercising, regardless of hair type, it's essential to refresh the hair as usual. This may involve reapplying styling products or lightly misting the hair with water to reactivate curls and enhance their definition. Choosing hair care products specifically formulated for curly, wavy, or coily hair types can help maintain moisture and prevent dryness, ensuring the curls remain healthy and vibrant even after intense workouts.

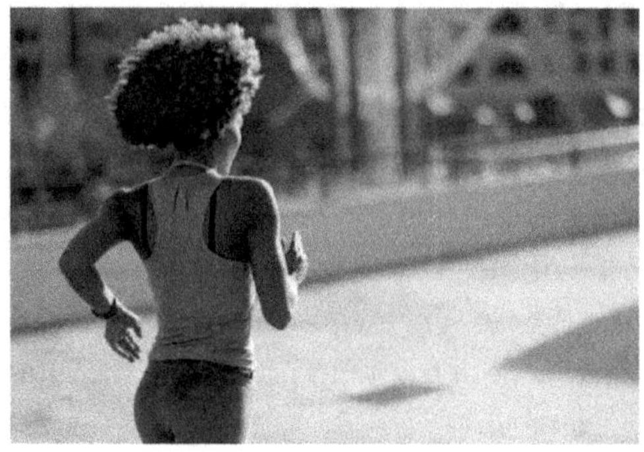

Incorporating these tips into your exercise and nighttime routine will undoubtedly play a significant role in preserving the longevity of your curly style. These small yet impactful adjustments ensure that your curls remain defined, frizz-free, and full of life throughout the day and into the night. By integrating these practices into your daily regimen, you can maintain the vibrancy and health of your curly hair for longer periods, allowing you to confidently showcase your natural beauty. Remember to choose the method that best suits your curl type and preferences to ensure optimal results.

9

Embracing Your Curly Hair

Love your curls fiercely. They're a part of what makes you, you.

Embracing curly hair extends far beyond mere aesthetics; it's a lifestyle that encompasses self-acceptance and celebration of natural beauty. For many, embracing curly hair marks a liberating journey of self-discovery and empowerment. Learning to care for your curly hair is an ongoing process, filled with trial and error, and experimentation. It's a journey of self-love and acceptance, where every curl is celebrated for its unique character and charm. Remember, caring for curly hair is a marathon, not a race. It requires patience, perseverance, and a willingness to embrace the natural rhythm and flow of your curls. So, as you embark on this journey, be kind to yourself, practice patience, and allow yourself the grace to embrace every twist and turn along the way. After all, each curl tells a story of beauty, resilience, and individuality.

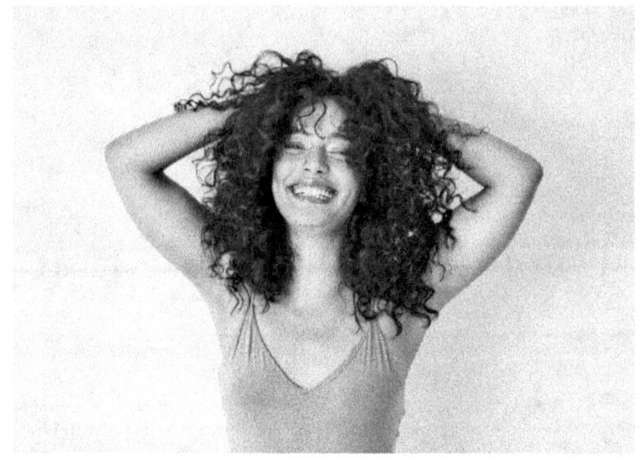

10

Product Guide

The following is a curated list of products that I've personally used and trusted, both on myself and in the salon. While these products have proven effective for me, it's important to recognize that everyone's hair is unique, and what works for one person may not necessarily work for another. Therefore, feel free to explore other options that may better suit your individual needs and preferences. The key is to find products that align with your hair type, concerns, and desired results, ensuring that your hair receives the care and nourishment it deserves.

Shampoos & Conditioners

- AG Balance Shampoo
- AG Boost Conditioner
- Aluram Moisturizing Shampoo
- Aluram Moisturizing Conditioner
- Aluram Purple Shampoo
- Aluram Volumizing Shampoo

- Aluram Volumizing Conditioner
- Amika Hydro Rush Intense Moisture Conditioner
- Innersense Color Awakening Hairbath
- Innersense Color Radiance Conditioner
- Innersense Hydrating Hairbath
- Innersense Hydrating Conditioner
- Uncle Funky's Daughter Squeaky Clean Shampoo
- Uncle Funky's Daughter Richee Rich Conditioner

Deep Conditioning

- Aluram Hydrate & Repair Mask
- Aluram Purple Hydrate & Repair Mask
- Amika Soulfood Nourishing Mask
- Amika The Kure Intense Bond Repair Mask
- Innersense Hydrating Hair Mask
- Olaplex No. 3 Hair Perfector

Foams/Mousses

- AG Care Mousse Gel
- Aluram Curl Foam
- Aluram Volumizing Foam
- The Doux Crazy Sexy Curl Foam
- The Doux Mousse Def Foam
- Innersense I Create Definition Styling Foam
- Innersense I Create Lift Volumizing Foam

Styling Gels

- Camille Rose Curl Maker
- Curl Mix Flaxseed Gel
- Innersense I Create Curl Memory
- Innersense I Create Hold
- Innersense I Create Volume
- Uncle Funky's Daughter Curly Magic

Finishing/Texture/Shine Sprays

- Aluram Dry Texture Spray
- Aluram Finishing Spray
- Aluram High Hold Finishing Spray

Finishing Oil

- Innersense I Create Shine
- Lanza Neem Plant Silk Scrum

11

Resources

Find a curl specialist in your area

DevaCut Stylist: https://www.devacurl.com/finder

Rezo Cut Stylist: https://rezoacademy.com/pages/store-locator-1

Cut It Kinky Tight Curl Specialist: https://www.cutitkinky.com/the-roster-1

Curl Magazine: https://readcurl.com/curlstylists/

My Style-List: https://mystyle-list.com/

12

About the Author

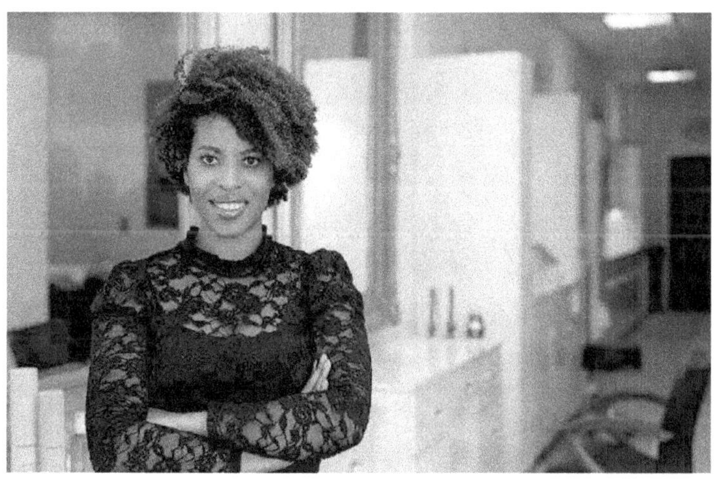

Ja'Nera Mitchom is a highly skilled and dedicated licensed cosmetologist with a specialized focus on curly hair, boasting eight years of expertise in the field. As the proud owner of Curls Unlimited salon in Roswell, GA, Ja'Nera has created a haven where clients can experience personalized care and embrace the beauty of their natural curls. Beyond her professional achievements, Ja'Nera is also a devoted single mom, balancing her passion for cosmetology with the joys and responsibilities of parenthood. Her commitment to excellence, both in her salon and in her personal life, sets her apart as a compassionate and talented professional within the industry.

http://www.janeranicole.com
http://facebook.com/janeranicole
http://www.instagram.com/curlsbyjaneranicole